CORTISOL FOR BEGINNERS

Empower Yourself With Insights And Strategies
To Navigate Cortisol Levels For Stress Hormone
Control, Optimal Health And Resilience

DR. ARIYA REYNA

CONTENTS

DISCLIAMER

This book is intended for informational purposes only and is not a substitute for professional medical advice, diagnosis, or treatment. The information provided in this book is based on the author's research and personal experiences and is not meant to replace the advice of healthcare professionals.

Readers are encouraged to consult with their healthcare providers before beginning any new exercise, wellness, or health program.

The author and publisher of this book are not responsible for any specific health or allergy needs that may require medical supervision and are not liable for any damages or negative consequences from any treatment, action, application, or preparation, to any person reading or following the information in this book.

The content of this book is not intended to be a substitute for professional medical advice, diagnosis, or treatment. Always seek the advice of your physician or other qualified health provider with any questions you may have regarding a medical condition.

The author and publisher disclaim responsibility for any adverse effects that may result from the use or application of the information contained in this book.

References to specific products, services, or organizations do not imply endorsement or recommendation by the author or the publisher.

The inclusion of such references is for illustrative purposes only. Thank you for reading and respecting the terms outlined in this disclaimer.

CHAPTER ONE

Cortisol: An Overview

Cortisol, sometimes known as the "stress hormone," is a vital steroid hormone generated by the adrenal glands located on top of each kidney. It is essential in many physiological processes and contributes to the general health of the organism. While cortisol is typically linked with stress, it is critical to realize its larger role in homeostasis maintenance.

Cortisol production has a diurnal pattern, with levels often rising in the early morning and falling in the late evening. This repetitive pattern is part of the body's natural circadian rhythm, which is controlled by light and dark cycles.

Cortisol's Function In The Body

Cortisol performs several roles that affect practically every system in the body. One of its key functions is to control metabolism by affecting fat, protein, and carbohydrate breakdown. Cortisol guarantees a continuous supply of energy during fasting or stress by increasing gluconeogenesis, the process of generating glucose from non-carbohydrate sources.

Cortisol also plays an important function in immune system modulation. It possesses anti-inflammatory characteristics, which assist the body in responding to and recovering from injuries or illnesses. A sustained increase in cortisol levels, on the other hand, might weaken the immune system, making the body more susceptible to illnesses.

Cortisol also influences bone development and maintenance by modulating calcium absorption in the intestines and bone reabsorption. Furthermore, it influences blood pressure and vascular tone, which is important for cardiovascular function.

Cortisol Levels Management

Cortisol levels are closely regulated by the hypothalamus-pituitary-adrenal (HPA) axis in response to numerous bodily signals. The hypothalamus initiates the process by generating corticotropin-releasing hormone (CRH).

This hormone stimulates the pituitary gland to create and release adrenocorticotropic hormone (ACTH), which causes the adrenal glands to produce and release cortisol.

Negative feedback mechanisms are critical in maintaining cortisol homeostasis. Cortisol levels rise, which inhibits the release of CRH and ACTH, resulting in less cortisol production. This feedback loop prevents excessive cortisol release and keeps the hormone at normal levels.

Cortisol's Functions

1. Metabolism Control:

Cortisol regulates macronutrient metabolism, guaranteeing a steady source of energy. It encourages gluconeogenesis, or the production of glucose from non-carbohydrate sources, and aids in the breakdown of lipids and proteins for energy.

2. Modulation of the Immune System:

Cortisol has anti-inflammatory as well as immunosuppressive properties. It aids the body's response to injuries or illnesses by reducing inflammation, but chronic increases might impair the immune system.

3. Health of the Bones:

Cortisol affects calcium absorption in the intestines as well as calcium reabsorption from bones. It is essential for bone growth and preservation.

4. Cardiovascular Performance:

The hormone affects blood pressure and vascular tone, which helps with cardiovascular health. Chronic elevation, on the other hand, might cause cardiovascular problems.

Stress And Cortisol

While cortisol is frequently connected with stress, understanding its role in the body's stress response is critical. The HPA axis is activated under stressful conditions, resulting in a rise in cortisol levels. This surge helps the body prepare for difficulties by mobilizing energy and increasing attentiveness.

Short-term cortisol elevations during acute stress are adaptive and aid the body in dealing with urgent dangers. Chronic stress, on the other hand, can cause permanent elevations in cortisol levels, which can be harmful to one's health.

The Consequences Of Chronic Cortisol Imbalance

1. Gaining Weight:

Prolonged cortisol rise is linked to increased belly fat accumulation. When paired with binge eating, this can result in weight gain and obesity.

2. Cognitive Function Impairment:

Cortisol levels that are chronically raised may impair cognitive function, impacting memory, focus, and decision-making. This is especially important in circumstances such as prolonged stress and certain mental health issues.

3. Sleep Disorders:

In the evening, cortisol levels normally decrease to encourage relaxation and sleep. However, chronic imbalance can disrupt this cycle, resulting in sleep disorders and insomnia.

4. Immune System Dysfunction:

While cortisol has anti-inflammatory qualities, long-term increases can weaken the immune system, making you more susceptible to infections and delaying recovery.

5. Cardiovascular Problems:

Long-term cortisol exposure may contribute to cardiovascular disorders such as hypertension and atherosclerosis.

6. Disorders of Mood:

Cortisol imbalances have been related to mood disorders such as sadness and anxiety. The precise relationship is complicated and varies from person to person.

Finally, cortisol is a complicated hormone that plays crucial functions in physiological homeostasis. While its connection to stress is well-known, it is critical to recognize its broader roles and the significance of maintaining a healthy cortisol balance. Chronic imbalances can affect metabolism, immunological function, cognitive health, and overall well-being.

Understanding the complicated interaction of cortisol in the body enables individuals to implement methods that maintain a balanced hormonal environment and boost overall health.

CHAPTER TWO

Understanding Cortisol And Its Effects For Beginners

The Cortisol-Hpa Axis

Cortisol is a steroid hormone generated by the adrenal glands on top of each kidney. It is essential for several human activities, including metabolic control, immunological response, and stress response. Cortisol's delicate link with the hypothalamic-pituitary-adrenal (HPA) axis is critical to understanding how this hormone affects human health.

The brain, pituitary gland, and adrenal glands are all involved in the HPA axis, which is a complicated feedback mechanism. When the body experiences physical or psychological stress, the hypothalamus releases corticotropin-releasing hormone (CRH). This hormone stimulates the pituitary gland to create and release adrenocorticotropic hormone (ACTH), which causes the adrenal glands to make and release cortisol into the circulation.

Cortisol is the body's major stress hormone, regulating different physiological processes in response to stress. It enhances alertness by mobilizing energy reserves, suppressing non-essential activities (such as the immune system and reproductive processes), and mobilizing energy reserves. While cortisol is necessary for life, persistent stress can disrupt the HPA axis, resulting in health problems such as adrenal exhaustion and metabolic diseases.

Cortisol Levels Analysis

Understanding cortisol levels is critical for measuring stress, recognizing potential health risks, and putting relevant measures in place. Cortisol levels have a diurnal regularity, increasing in the early morning and falling after midnight. Cortisol levels are measured using a variety of ways, including blood tests, saliva testing, and urine tests.

Blood tests are routinely used in clinical settings to obtain a snapshot of cortisol levels at a certain time.

Cortisol levels, however, can change throughout the day, and a single blood test may not provide an accurate picture. Saliva tests, on the other hand, provide a more thorough picture by assessing cortisol levels throughout the day. Salivary cortisol testing is non-invasive and may be performed at home, making it an ideal choice for tracking diurnal rhythms.

Urine tests reveal cortisol metabolites and give a more comprehensive evaluation of cortisol production over 24 hours. This approach is beneficial for assessing total cortisol production and finding diurnal rhythm anomalies. Each testing technique has benefits, and the method of choosing is determined by the specific information required for diagnosis or monitoring.

Natural Cortisol Management

Cortisol level regulation is critical for general health since persistent elevation or depletion can lead to health problems. Fortunately, some lifestyle changes can help you control cortisol naturally:

1. Techniques for Stress Management: Meditation, deep breathing, and yoga can trigger the body's relaxation response, reducing the influence of stress on cortisol levels.

2. Adequate Sleep: Adequate sleep is required to maintain a healthy diurnal cortisol cycle. Creating a suitable sleep environment and sticking to a regular sleep pattern will help lower cortisol levels.

3. Regular Physical exercise: Regular physical exercise can assist in normalizing cortisol levels. However, strong or continuous activity, especially if not followed by proper recuperation, may temporarily raise cortisol levels. Finding a happy medium is essential.

4. Healthy eating habits, such as fruits, vegetables, and whole grains, contribute to general well-being and may impact cortisol management. Excessive coffee and processed sweets should also be avoided.

5. Maintaining healthy social ties and a support system can help lessen feelings of isolation and

stress, which has a favorable influence on cortisol levels.

6. Mindfulness and Relaxation: Including mindfulness activities in your everyday life, such as progressive muscle relaxation or guided imagery, can help you relax and regulate your cortisol levels.

7. Hydration: Dehydration is a stressor for the body that can impact cortisol levels. Getting enough water is a simple yet effective method to improve overall health.

Cortisol-Related Medical Conditions

While cortisol is required for regular physiological function, abnormalities can result in several medical disorders. Among these conditions are:

1. Cushing's Syndrome: Cushing's syndrome is characterized by extended exposure to high amounts of cortisol. It can be caused by adrenal tumors, long-term use of corticosteroid drugs, or excessive ACTH synthesis by the pituitary gland.

2. Addison's disease, on the other hand, develops when the adrenal glands fail to generate enough cortisol and aldosterone. This disease can be caused by autoimmune illnesses, infections, or other conditions that cause adrenal gland injury.

3. Adrenal Fatigue: While not widely recognized as a medical illness, adrenal fatigue is frequently connected with chronic stress and is thought to be caused by continuous periods of high cortisol, resulting in exhaustion, sleep problems, and other symptoms.

4. Post-Traumatic Stress Disorder (PTSD): People suffering from PTSD may have dysregulation of the HPA axis, resulting in elevated cortisol levels. This hormone imbalance is likely to contribute to the disorder's emotional and physiological symptoms.

Cortisol And Rest

Cortisol and sleep have a complicated interaction that is important for general health. Cortisol levels normally follow a diurnal cycle, spiking in the early morning to encourage wakefulness and falling over the night to allow for restorative sleep. Disruptions in this rhythm, on the other hand, can influence sleep quality and contribute to sleep disorders.

Chronic stress, which contributes significantly to high cortisol levels, can interfere with the ability to fall and maintain asleep. As previously stated, stress management strategies can be very effective in managing this condition. Individuals suffering from disorders such as insomnia or sleep apnea may also have abnormal cortisol rhythms.

Adequate sleep is necessary for maintaining a healthy cortisol cycle, while cortisol levels, on the other hand, can impact sleep quality. Sleep difficulties may be exacerbated by disruptions to the normal cortisol cycle, such as those noticed in shift workers or persons with irregular sleep patterns. Setting a consistent sleep schedule, developing a calming nighttime ritual, and improving sleep hygiene are all critical for ensuring healthy cortisol levels and quality sleep.

To summarize, knowing cortisol and its different aspects is critical for those seeking to improve their health and well-being. A complete approach can contribute to a balanced hormonal profile and improved general health, from the complicated interplay with the HPA axis to detecting cortisol levels and adopting natural management measures. Furthermore, understanding the relationship between cortisol and sleep emphasizes the need to develop appropriate sleep patterns for a harmonious and well-functioning body.

CHAPTER THREE

Understanding Cortisol's Role In Exercise For Beginners

Cortisol is an important hormone generated by the adrenal glands that is frequently related to stress reactions. When it comes to exercise, however, cortisol plays a more complicated role in the body. Understanding this hormone and its association with physical exercise is critical for novices who want to improve their fitness routines.

Exercise, whether aerobic or weight training, raises cortisol levels. This surge serves various functions, including delivering a fast energy boost to the body and decreasing inflammation. Cortisol, in modest doses, is advantageous for the body's stress response, assisting in muscle repair and recovery.

However, prolonged or severe activity might result in chronically high cortisol levels, which can be harmful. Cortisol levels that are too high might lead to muscle protein breakdown and inhibit muscular development. It may also weaken the immune system and increase the likelihood of injury. To avoid cortisol excess, it is critical to find a balance between exercise intensity and duration.

Furthermore, the timing of exercise might affect cortisol levels. Morning exercises frequently coincide with the natural cortisol peak, which can improve exercise performance. Intense nighttime exercises, on the other hand, may alter the body's normal cortisol pattern, thereby impacting sleep quality.

The goal for novices is to engage in a well-rounded workout plan that incorporates aerobic, strength, and flexibility training. This method lowers cortisol levels while improving general health and fitness.

Cortisol With Nutrition For Beginners

Nutrition is important in managing cortisol levels, and knowing the link between the two is critical for those just starting on their wellness path. Cortisol, widely known as the "stress hormone," reacts to both psychological and dietary stressors.

Balanced and healthy meals help to regulate cortisol levels. Consuming a diet rich in whole foods, such as fruits and vegetables, whole grains, and lean meats, for example, supplies the body with vital nutrients that promote adrenal function. Adequate hydration is also important since dehydration can cause cortisol release.

Furthermore, the time and nature of meals affect cortisol levels. Spreading meals out throughout the day helps to keep blood sugar levels constant and prevents cortisol increases linked with energy dumps. Incorporating complex carbs, healthy fats, and proteins into each meal promotes a more balanced hormonal response, supporting long-term energy and emotional stability.

Excessive intake of refined sugars and processed meals, on the other hand, might cause blood sugar swings and cortisol release.

Caffeine, which is typically present in energy drinks and coffee, can also raise cortisol levels. As a result, newcomers should be cautious about their dietary choices, preferring a nutrient-dense and well-balanced diet.

Furthermore, proper sleep is essential for cortisol management. Sleep deprivation can upset the body's hormonal balance, resulting in heightened cortisol levels and greater vulnerability to stress.

 A cortisol-friendly lifestyle requires establishing a regular sleep regimen and generating a pleasant sleeping environment.

To assist cortisol management, beginners should focus on a nutrient-dense diet, sufficient hydration, and excellent sleep hygiene. These lifestyle choices influence not just cortisol levels but also general well-being.

The Effects Of Cortisol On Mental Health: A Beginner's Guide

Cortisol, well recognized for its function in the body's stress response, also has an impact on mental health. It is critical for newcomers seeking a deeper grasp of this link to appreciate the complicated interplay between cortisol and the brain.

Cortisol is produced in reaction to stress to mobilize energy and improve attentiveness. While this is an adaptive reaction in the short term, persistent exposure to increased cortisol levels can be damaging to mental health. Anxiety, sadness, and poor cognitive performance have all been related to elevated cortisol levels.

Understanding stress management tactics is critical for beginners trying to reduce cortisol's influence on mental health. Regular physical activity, mindfulness techniques like meditation and deep breathing, and social support can all assist in controlling cortisol levels and enhance emotional well-being. A balanced diet, enough sleep, and time spent in nature are also important components of a holistic approach to mental wellness.

Beginners should be aware of the symptoms of chronic stress and cortisol dysregulation, such as persistent sensations of worry or exhaustion. Seeking expert help from healthcare doctors or mental health professionals might give useful insights and assistance.

Cortisol And Aging: A Beginner's Guide

Cortisol's involvement in the body becomes more important as people age. Cortisol, which is frequently connected with stress, can influence several elements of the aging process. Understanding the impacts of cortisol on aging is critical for novices navigating this complicated connection to make educated wellness decisions.

The effect of cortisol on muscle mass is one important factor. Cortisol levels that are elevated, particularly in reaction to persistent stress, can lead to muscle protein breakdown and muscle mass loss. Catabolism is a worry for aging people because it may contribute to sarcopenia or age-related loss in muscle mass and function.

Cortisol is also tightly tied to the body's inflammatory response. While inflammation is a normal and important aspect of the immune system, chronic inflammation associated with high cortisol levels has been linked to age-related illnesses such as cardiovascular disease, diabetes, and neurodegenerative disorders.

Stress management through lifestyle modifications becomes critical as novices approach their older years. Exercise, including both aerobic and resistance training, can help control cortisol levels and prevent muscle loss. Additionally, stress-reduction methods such as meditation, yoga, and appropriate sleep are becoming increasingly crucial for general health maintenance.

Nutritional choices also play an important role in cortisol regulation as people become older. A diet high in antioxidants and anti-inflammatory foods, such as fruits, vegetables, and omega-3 fatty acids, can help reverse cortisol's aging effects.

Finally, newcomers should be aware of the complex link between cortisol and aging. Adopting a comprehensive approach that includes stress management, regular exercise, and a nutrient-dense diet can all help to promote good aging and well-being.

Understanding Cortisol's Impact On Immune Function For Beginners

Cortisol is a key hormone generated by the adrenal glands that play an important function in many physiological processes in the body. One of its most important jobs is to impact immunological function. Cortisol has a complicated function in modulating immunological responses, which is the body's defensive mechanism against infections.

Cortisol has anti-inflammatory and immunosuppressive properties. When under stress, the body produces more cortisol, which helps to suppress the immunological response. While this suppression may be advantageous in the short term, persistent cortisol rise, as observed with prolonged stress, may have a deleterious impact on immunological function.

Cortisol's immunosuppressive effects are mostly due to a decrease in immune cell activation. Lymphocytes and monocytes are white blood cells that are crucial components of the immune system. Cortisol suppresses the formation and function of these cells, leaving the body more vulnerable to infection.

Cortisol's anti-inflammatory effects, on the other hand, aid in the prevention of excessive inflammation in response to stress. Inflammation is a normal and important aspect of the immune response, but it can cause a variety of health problems if it becomes chronic. Cortisol reduces inflammation by decreasing the production of pro-inflammatory chemicals like cytokines.

It is vital to highlight that the effect of cortisol on immunological function is a delicate balance. While acute cortisol rises under stress might temporarily inhibit the immune system from allocating resources to more urgent dangers, persistent cortisol elevations may harm long-term immunological function. As a result, stress management and the use of appropriate coping methods are critical for maintaining a healthy immune system.

CHAPTER FOUR

The Balancing Act Of Cortisol And Inflammation

Inflammation is a normal and required immune system reaction to damage or illness. Chronic inflammation, on the other hand, can lead to the development of a variety of health issues, including autoimmune illnesses, cardiovascular diseases, and metabolic disorders. Cortisol is a double-edged sword when it comes to controlling inflammation.

Cortisol has significant anti-inflammatory characteristics that aid in the resolution of inflammation after the immune system has dealt with the initial assault.

It accomplishes this by preventing the creation and release of pro-inflammatory chemicals such as cytokines and prostaglandins. This anti-inflammatory activity is critical for preventing severe and protracted inflammation, which can cause tissue damage.

While cortisol's anti-inflammatory properties are critical for health, chronic cortisol increase, which is commonly linked with long-term stress, can upset this delicate balance.

Prolonged exposure to high amounts of cortisol may result in glucocorticoid resistance, a condition in which the body becomes less receptive to cortisol's anti-inflammatory properties. This can lead to chronic inflammation and a higher risk of inflammatory illnesses.

Furthermore, cortisol's role in inflammation is not limited to its direct anti-inflammatory actions. It also communicates with other hormonal systems, such as the sympathetic nervous system, which influences the overall inflammatory response.

Understanding and regulating stress levels is therefore critical for maintaining a healthy cortisol response and avoiding chronic inflammation.

The Stress-Weight Connection In Cortisol And Weight Management

Cortisol and weight control have a complicated interaction that includes several physiological mechanisms. Cortisol is known as the "stress hormone," and its levels rise in reaction to a variety of stresses, both physical and psychological. This stress-induced increase in cortisol has various implications for weight management.

One important component is cortisol's influence on energy metabolism regulation. Cortisol increases the mobilization of energy stores under stressful conditions, resulting in an enhanced release of glucose into the circulation. This is part of the body's "fight or flight" reaction, which provides a rapid supply of energy to respond to imminent dangers. Chronic stress, on the other hand, might result in chronically high cortisol levels, which contribute to glucose overproduction and, as a result, insulin resistance.

Insulin resistance, a disease in which cells become less receptive to insulin's actions, can lead to fat buildup, particularly around the belly. This visceral fat in the abdomen is linked to an elevated risk of metabolic illnesses such as type 2 diabetes and cardiovascular disease.

Furthermore, persistent stress and high cortisol levels may impact dietary choices and appetites. During stressful times, many people have an increased appetite for high-calorie, sweet, and fatty meals. This can lead to overeating and the consumption of unhealthy foods, wreaking havoc on weight control.

Adopting stress-reduction methods such as regular exercise, proper sleep, and mindfulness practices can help to reduce the effects of cortisol on weight control. These lifestyle changes not only assist in reducing cortisol levels but also contribute to general well-being and a healthier weight.

Cortisol And Hormonal Balance: Endocrine System Navigation

Hormonal balance is essential for appropriate bodily function since it influences different physiological processes such as metabolism, development, and reproduction. As a steroid hormone, cortisol interacts with and impacts the activity of other hormones in the endocrine system, resulting in a complex regulatory dance.

Cortisol and sex hormones, notably estrogen and testosterone, have a significant connection. Chronic stress and high cortisol levels can affect sex hormone balance, resulting in irregular menstrual cycles, reduced libido, and reproductive concerns in both men and women. Furthermore, cortisol might compete with sex hormones for receptor binding sites, impairing their overall activity.

Cortisol also interacts with thyroid hormones, which play an important role in metabolic regulation. High cortisol levels can decrease thyroid gland activity, resulting in a condition known as "thyroid suppression," which can cause symptoms such as weariness, weight gain, and sluggish metabolism.

Furthermore, cortisol impacts insulin synthesis, a hormone involved in blood sugar regulation. Chronic cortisol rise can cause insulin resistance, impair glucose metabolism, and increase the risk of type 2 diabetes.

The maintenance of hormonal balance is critical for general health and well-being. Stress management, regular exercise, a balanced diet, and appropriate sleep are all strategies to enhance hormonal equilibrium. These lifestyle variables contribute not just to cortisol management but also to total endocrine system homeostasis.

To summarize, knowing the role of cortisol in immunological function, inflammation, weight control, and hormonal balance is critical for novices looking to comprehend the complexity of this important hormone. While cortisol performs important purposes in the body's response to stress, keeping a healthy cortisol level is critical to avoiding potential health consequences. Implementing stress-reduction lifestyle measures, such as regular exercise, proper sleep, and mindfulness practices, can lead to a healthier cortisol profile and general well-being.

Conclusion

To summarize, knowing cortisol is critical for general well-being since this hormone plays a vital part in the body's stress response. "Cortisol for Beginners" provides an in-depth examination of this hormone's actions, regulation, and influence on many body systems. Readers now understand how cortisol, which is generated by the adrenal glands, regulates metabolism, immunological function, and the circadian rhythm of the body.

The guidance highlights the necessity of maintaining a healthy cortisol level, as both excess and shortage can cause health problems. It gives practical insights into lifestyle issues such as stress management, appropriate sleep, and regular exercise that can either alleviate or worsen cortisol levels. With this information, novices may make educated decisions to promote a healthy cortisol balance.

Furthermore, "Cortisol for Beginners" emphasizes the mind-body connection, shedding attention to the interconnection of mental and physical wellness. Recognizing the influence of stress on cortisol secretion enables people to take a more holistic approach to their well-being.

By the end of this primer, readers will have gained an essential understanding to navigate the complex function of cortisol in their daily lives, boosting resilience and vitality.

THE END